swirl

by
constance bacchus

<u>acknowledgements</u>

Thank you to Figroot Press who first published 'finding the storm before it arrives on the top of cascade hill' when the author's name was constance schultz

& thank you to Feral: A Journal of Poetry and Art for first publishing 'the wind has started/ oh she is'.

this book is dedicated to the storms in washington state
and the people who enjoy them

mirror

rock pigeons & osprey young
gaze over at midway
avenue occasionally
cats from north dam
park there may be more
cats in this town than
people it's a shame it's
empty it's a weekend dogs
precocious & friendly scout
for action order a beer
it's all summer lawnmowers
helicopters basketball down
the way beginning to cool must
be evening cars track shadows
shifting deep air thick w/things
inappropriate to mention in this heat

finding the storm before it arrives on the top of cascade
hill

cotton balls in the
sky
unthreading

the lake as slate
rolls rough arches
beneath a low thundercloud

voices carry
up
excitement at
the park

bending trees
once forgotten picnic tables
& a girl
running creating her own wind

the shallows ooze muddy
with shadows
swimming

& a light glorious paints the trees

outside electric city

frozen movements in the bay
in clouds rolling
down the wall
fast

boaters notice

pop music distractions
pictures of fish
all of the lake

half-lidded eyes
& beat w/o a guitar

half the valley
storms far away
on both sides
& what's
coming

did it stop even

what rages on
the way to omak
to soap lake

what dancing god
random visits
wilbur & bridgeport

firecracker coulee blue

I hear something
& my breath
catches

I hear a robin
imitate
a laser

see a jet streak

harbingers

uneven air of the coulee
rides smoke down the channel

lashes & plays
hiding the heat

blows dust eddies

blows dried up leaves
in summer until fresh

mown lawns
seem unused wild & full
of snakes

her breath whistles harsh
tickles out of the ear

rustles & clangs
on flagpoles

& I wonder about the spirits carried

the wind has started/oh she is

started she blows warmer
in your ears than she looks
envelopes/ bemoans you
she has all these/ let your hair
ideas because they/ fly

the sun is out & favorite weeds
you know how she gets/ do you see
about shadows/ the island
I love you/she stops/ through your
coffee no sugar describing/ she is

waiting somewhere in 2
words, on a 2 lane, a thousand

no chill, she is swirling, can you
walk to the water/ one ear looking up
& the other just alkaline/polite, listen, soft
aches/she misses you/she is ringing
chimes in the neighbor's yard/ the cemetery

remembering & she stands at the beginning of the lake,
looks north & thinks of all the people there past the rocks/
feels the sun brush soft/ the water in the air/she feels the
walk itself/ the flight of the clouds/beautiful/
structured hills/ the cuts of the sides like acres of
chocolate

stories the wind tells

erratically placed along the
canal boulders rise

in clumps in families
& that's how they should

be on hot days in the desert
bickering w/hawks aglide

red-tailed hawks looking
for ravens to wrestle or
avoid looking for rattlers

outstretched badger on a
tall pile of rocks hands
on hips

tsk tsk daring a
confrontation anytime

can't hear music w/doors propped open
echoes on the other side can't see

anything but mule deer grazing

do you have rain today or wish you did

do you ever pray   on stormy days
for rain to fall   tears fall
upon waters in coulees   kiss

to flood   on sunlight streaming
caves/tucked away   just kiss
to seize summer heat   meander wander over

rain to whisper   leave a trace
at desert rocks   no copse
to water sage   clouds roll
autonomous raven   breeze

so wet see/ barely feel
grey & green/ melancholy holds
smoky fire in mountains   no lake scatter

does the ocean even know   love w/care

pool in middle of dry summer city
warm w/rain/rain & lips painted
expose to flash from sky

to say that   on a morning in
december
                                  ice on the ground
                                  & snow

rain just begins w/water & that wicked magic

an interactive element of earth culture
art of nature much despised

a familiar element in seattle
promoting nostalgia
in that salespeak
pushes
entices
ordinary people away from
technology

a rapture of green
blue
sad
rattling w/a mixture of wet hair

look
wake up
cold

rain climbing down your neck
that should do it

texting someone up the canyon 30 miles away during a
storm

rain in arlington is different
than in central washington
heavier happens all the time
grey sky grey rain grey thoughts
no shadows here there is a
brilliant sun that rises from
the dam paints the water blue
deep in dark weather & it is
tinted w/ electricity thunder
perhaps it is displayed in certain
places for miles where it is not
raining yet & won't for half an
hour from now

on hearing voices in the dark during a blackout

if you make the rain your friend
then it's okay
when the power is gone

(electricity
computers
phones)

you can listen
to large wet drops
fall into a puddle
off the gutter

caught in a window-well
caught

& it marches
does not absorb
those drops

I hear repeat
crystal clear clean
rain

carrying voices of something
that shouldn't be out at night
bothering people
in the dark
rain

flooding

the rain has voices
i can almost
understand what they say

something about sleep
& time
drops like a leaky roof

the rain sounds like
it is flooding in skagit
even though we are here

& it echoes of sandbags
every year

every year
every flood
an emergency

to be planned
over whiskey
at the legion
when avoiding
police on the way home

written by candlelight when the power went out

the rain is just the rain
the dark is just that

the dark & the rain
& water
throws itself
out of the way
displaced
on valley road

& the rain
sounds dark
& heavy
but steady as a heartbeat

even in the total night
it keeps the beat
not afraid
of who can brcak in
when the power goes out
that's the rain for you
dependable & wet
echoes in the ears

louder when sound is all you can see
louder until it's all
& so loud builds itself a lake
w/secrets folded in the waves

rain in the window-well of a cinderblock house

rain, clear w/some dirt
not smelling of car oil, nail polish

rain, could be from the lake or dam
w/o salmon, in the window-well watching

rain, it colors, reflects
it goes to the coast & stays awhile

& sometimes can be seen in soap lake
if lucky at the park

rain can't compete w/candles
although it lasts longer

& dark, the dark will be there after the rain is gone

the atmosphere of flying magical in the water

rain
falls
on
the
water

rain
drops
drop
ping
sing

((songs))

&
rain
sounds
the same on
the ocean pacific
as pike place market

whether orcas or humans
occasionally stop to   listen

...& does not care where they are going you look so lovely
in the rain that is because it makes my hair curl rain mist
raindrops rain rain go away keep falling on my head
rainbows flooding waters up walls of rain fall down & does
not care where they are going...

trail at northrup point

through the trees
& berry bushes
w/crimson fruit
the blue lake peaks

& trail is dry remembering
an invincible pulaski
friends all the weeds are far enough &

forgetful blue at the end
is not so framed
expands w/ reeds
bending to the water

& if you do not
get your hair wet
heat catches
you & windows
down all the way home

the end

<u>notes</u>

about the author

Constance Bacchus was born in central Washington state and now resides there with her daughter. She has a fondness for nature and will often accompany her to local parks.

The writing of Ms Bacchus has appeared in literary magazines far and wide, most recently in Cats & Dogs Reigning, Salmon Creek Journal, Train, Cathexis Northwest and Them Dam Writers Online.

constance bacchus
po box 374
coulee city, wa 99115
conniebacchus@yahoo.com

www.ingramcontent.com/pod-product-compliance
Lightning Source LLC
Chambersburg PA
CBHW051410250726
48656CB00006B/2376